Healthy Living Secrets

10 Habits for a Healthier Next Year

Stephanie L. Zahl

WorkwithStephanieZahl.com

Zahl Family Publishing

Note to Readers

This book contains the opinions and experiences of the author. It is for informational purposes only. The information given here is to help you make informed decisions about your health. The reader should consult a medical professional before adopting any of the suggestions in this book. The author/publisher disclaims all responsibility for any use of this book or the materials within.

Liability Disclaimer

By reading this document, you assume all risks associated with using the advice given below, with a full understanding that you, solely, are responsible for anything that may occur as a result of putting this information into action in any way, and regardless of your interpretation of the advice.

Terms of Use

You are given a non-transferable, "personal use" license to this product. You cannot distribute it or share it with other individuals.

Also, there are no resale rights or private label rights granted when purchasing this document. In other words, it's for your own personal use only.

Contents

Introduction

Do you ever feel like keeping your family healthy shouldn't be this difficult? I know I do. Maybe good health just requires a little offense instead of always being on the defense. Maybe you could use a game plan.

Do you seem to have the same health problems at almost the same time every year? Think about it. There is Flu Season, Allergy Season, Hay Fever Season, and Cold Season. The fact that something is labeled a season should give you a chance to prepare.

I can tell you when patients are going to have a cold, or an allergy based on the calendar. We all know it. Why do you think the stores move what you are going to need for each season to the front row?

The last time I went to the store I noticed all the allergy medications had been moved to a special rack. That's probably a better indication of spring in Michigan than our state bird the Robin coming home.

I can't believe how many of my patients come in completely surprised by their health conditions, even though they experience the same ones year after year. I have one patient I'm waiting for who will come in worried that she's getting a cold any day now. She will have herself on every cold medication she can, and be complaining that her MD won't let her have any Antibiotics. She has a good doctor thank goodness. In a couple of weeks she will figure out its allergies, and order our allergy vitamins, and presto it will be all better. Think about the money and aggravation she could save herself if she would just plan ahead.

The whole system of waiting until something goes wrong to fix it is driving me a little crazy. So I decided to be a little more proactive. I went through a pile of our patient's charts trying to figure out what problems we address every year.

In this simple guide, I'm giving you the information we give our patients year after year. These are the tricks we use at home to take care of our family. Something as simple as adding lemon to your water can make a huge difference. I hope the advice contained in this book helps you take care of your family so you can get through the yearly yucks.

New Year, New You

New Year is time to think about your health again. I don't know about you, but after pigging out during the Holidays my mind turns to weight loss. In fact I think we all know what the most popular New Year's resolution is weight loss. I read a stat last year that said 80% of people's New Year's resolutions involve weight loss, exercise, or both. I'm not sure how they know what resolutions people are making, but judging by what we see in our office I'd say 80% is a good guess.

I'm going to talk about something that can cause you to lose weight, but it's really not what I'm going to focus on. My husband and I start every year with a fast. We feel that it helps us get the year off on the right foot health wise.

Are you imagining wandering around lost in the wilderness for 40 days with nothing to eat? That's not what I'm talking about. There are a lot of different ways to fast. Think about Lent. Lent is a form of fasting. You might not be religious, so maybe you are unfamiliar with lent, but I think most people have at least heard of it. You don't have to be a Catholic to look forward to getting paczki's from the store before Lent.

Fasting is removing something from your diet. It could be coffee, meat, pop, anything. Now if you are religious, most religions embrace a form a fasting in their faith. You could look into that angle and see what would be appropriate for you.

The fast we choose is the Daniel Fast, which is eating only fruits and vegetables for three weeks along with just water to drink. While we do fast for spiritual reasons as well, the main purpose is to clean our bodies of as many toxins as possible, to do that we eat the purest and least processed foods we can.

The Daniel fast is one of the easiest fasts to do. I recommend that you buy Jentezen Franklin's book on fasting, or go online to find directions on how to do it. I recommend picking one site that makes the most sense to you and following that one.

You have a chance at the beginning of every year to clean up your body. The best thing about starting in January is that you don't look weird to everyone around you, because they are all working on their New Year's resolutions too.

The other thing about starting in January is its right after the holidays. If you are like most people, you have been living on goodies since November. When January arrives you feel fat and terrible.

There is nothing like the feeling you get when you know you are starting a new year out with a body you took the time to tune up. Cleaning the toxins out of your body is like cleaning the sludge out of your engine. Everything runs better when it's done, allowing your body to deal better with the challenges of a new year.

Action Steps

1. If your doctor says you are healthy enough try a fast. There is a lot of information online about how to fast. Look up something that you think you can do and start from there. It doesn't have to be anything extensive just start small and work your way up.

Choose one day a week that you don't eat meat, or skip the pop for the day. We prefer to do a Daniel fast. Google Daniel Fast if that sounds interesting to you. I will tell you what I tell my kids," Just do, no excuses choose something and do it."

The Winter Blues

It's February in West Michigan. Choose an answer to guess how I can tell?

1. I haven't seen even a glimmer of the sun in almost 2 weeks.

2. it's really, really cold.

3. it's wet and nasty.

4. All my patients are tired and grumpy.

If you chose any of the answers above you are right. I think everyone around here suffers at least a little from Seasonal Depression. I know I used to.

   Winter has always been a trial for me. There is just something almost oppressive about winter in West Michigan, you feel this weight on you and you just can't get on top of it.

   For years I couldn't get on top of it. I was suffering from Fibromyalgia. I was tired and in pain all the time add to that dealing with seasonal depression I was miserable. The combination was exhausting and I slept all the time. I missed a lot of time with my children because of my illness, time I will never get back.

It took years of work and research before I finally found ways to control my fibromyalgia. The fibromyalgia is actually one of the reasons I believe so strongly in fasting and detox. If I don't regularly clean out my body, I relapse.

I know for many of us the winter blues is a culmination of other issues, but we believe this list will still do you some good.

Here is the list of what we recommend to our patients who are suffering from the winter blues.

1. Get a full spectrum light of some kind. I know it won't replace the sun, but it does seem to take the edge off for a lot of our patients. I recommend having it right in your bathroom. That way you can have it on you while you are getting ready in the morning.

Some people claim that if you sit under it naked it helps more. I don't know if that's right, but if you are going to be sitting around naked the bathroom would be a good place to do it.

2. Drink green tea. Green tea is known to be an anti-depressant. So we recommend it to our patients, and it does seem to help. We love green tea and recommend it to everyone. I will talk more about green tea later.

3. Eat turmeric. If you like Indian food stock up, turmeric is a spice traditionally found in Indian cuisine. It is also known to have anti-depressant tendencies. We eat a lot of turmeric in our cooking, and I didn't even notice a blip of my

moodiness this year. If you think you don't like Indian food you can get it in a pill form, or it is really good in chicken soup, something else that has been proven to help you feel better.

4. Take your B vitamins; B's are the best stress relief in the world. When my husband was in school he worked at a volunteer clinic that had several alcoholic patients. My husband convinced a couple of them to try B-vitamins, and the results were amazing.
   We believe the alcohol strips the body of all its B-vitamins leaving you unable to deal with any stress. We think that is why alcoholics end up like they do. They just can't deal with anything and the bottle keeps them numb so they don't have to. When I got depressed in the winter that was how I felt, and I know there are days when Marty feels that way. A couple of B-vitamins and all is right with the world.

5. Okay I'm mentioning D-vitamins only so you don't say why didn't she mention D-vitamins? We have all been told that's what you need for the winter blues, and you do need them. I'm just hoping you are already taking them so you don't need to hear it from me. The single best source of D-vitamins is Sunlight 15 minutes on the face and arms daily. If you do decide to supplement your D's make sure they are not synthetic.

6. Personally I also like to drink a lot of orange juice when I can in the winter. I'm not sure if it's because it makes me think of a warm place or if it's all the vitamin C but it makes me feel better.

When you drink orange juice get unsweetened you do not need the extra sugar they put in orange juice.

Action Steps

1. Get a full spectrum light. Go to Lowes or another hardware store and see what they have, before you buy an expensive one. Of course if there is one you really love get it.

2. Get a good B-vitamin. You want your vitamin to have all the B's in it. We recommend getting Cataplex B and Cataplex G from Standard Process together they make a full B complex.

3. Drink green tea after dinner every night. This is one of the least expensive ways you can improve your health.

4. Try some Indian food. There are a lot of good recipes online. As well as some really good premade versions available at most grocery stores.

5. Vitamin C is a good pick me up, and it's great for your immune system. Fresh oranges and grapefruits are an excellent way to start your day.

Why are you so tired?

Unfortunately, this is one we can't answer without your medical history. It could be low thyroid, adrenal fatigue, low testosterone, etc. There are a lot of choices and without the proper information I can't help you as much as I'd like. Now that we've got that out of the way there are some simple choices you can make that may make a difference.

Sorry to all you evening couch potatoes, but you need to turn off the TV. Apparently the TV causes reactions in your mind and body that may keep you from getting a good night's sleep. I know you think you are relaxing, but according to studies you aren't.

Read a fiction book for an hour before bed, instead of watching TV. Don't do what I've been doing and try to learn something right before bed. I don't retain it, or my mind spends the whole night trying to figure it out.

Go to bed at the same time every night. I can't tell you how much better I feel when I do that. If you can I recommend a 10 PM bed time it seems to work best with most people's body rhythms.

Don't think you can catch up on sleep on the weekend in the long run that just doesn't work.

I know some of us can't shut off our minds. When I have a night like that I take valerian root. Valerian root is the natural alternative to Valium.

While valerian is not considered physically addictive, you can become mentally addicted to it if you think you have to use it every night. I only take it for up to a week at a time and not on the weekends.

It works really well if I can't sleep because of pain. Valerian will make you very sleepy so you can't take it for pain relief during the day. I recommend taking it a half hour to fifteen minutes before bed if you've had a bad day and don't think you will be able to sleep. If you take it too early you will miss the best time to use it for falling asleep.

On the other end of the bedtime problem you also want to get up at about the same time every day. I know it's not something you want to do on the weekends, but if you start to feel better it's worth it.

Don't eat sugar 3 hours before bed time. (My husband say's ice cream is especially bad.) This seems to cause weird dreams and restlessness in a lot of people. Just think about kids after a birthday party or Halloween. My husband could give you the biology and chemistry behind it, but it's easier to just avoid it.

You need to move every day. People don't move like they used to. Our lives have gotten pretty sedentary. My job and probably yours is mostly sitting. We have gone from people that work in the fields to people that sit behind computer desks all day. These changes make it harder to get the exercise we need.

One simple change you can make to get a bit more movement in is to stand when you are working, it is good for you and it makes you sound more positive and energetic when you are on the phone. I like to stand up right before I answer the phone or make a phone call as weird as it seems the people on the other end can feel it.

Now if you're like me you will try to move when your kids can't see you, and mock you. The old fashioned calisthenics from gym class are great. If you live somewhere that walking is possible do it.

Keep things simple add a little more movement to your life every week. It is easy to keep doing little things, trying to rearrange your life to get to the gym is not.

Action Steps

1. Turn off the TV you are probably just stressing yourself out.

2. Set and keep a bed time and wake up time apparently a schedule is good for you.

3. Try valerian on rough nights it should help you settle and get some rest. There is research that shows a chemical pattern that stops some people from sleeping. Our patients have had good results with the valerian.

4. Move your body in some way every day as little as 5 minutes of exercise daily can make a huge difference. Any amount of exercise is better than no exercise.
.

5. No sugary treats in the 3 hours before bed, try to limit your fluid intake too. Nothing ruins a great dream like having to go to the bathroom.

Spring Allergies

April showers bring May allergies. I love spring the whole world comes alive again. The flowers are blooming, the trees are budding, and there is pollen everywhere.

Growing up I lived in a complete haze. I was always full of Benadryl. From the time the grass started to show through the snow until the snows covered it up again. I was allergic to everything.

Through a lot of testing on me the official guinea pig we found vitamins that almost completely get rid of my allergies. We have shared these vitamins with a lot of our patients always with good results.

Now you can only get these vitamins from a Chiropractor, but if you go online or call the company they can help you find someone who carries them. The company is called Standard Process and they are out of Wisconsin go to www.standardprocess.com to find a doctor near you.

Allerplex is what we use for stopping allergies before they start. Most of the time the allerplex is enough, but when it's not we use Antronex.

Antronex is for those super strong allergies. We actually use it for poison ivy. I give it to my family as soon as I know they were exposed. Sometimes it's not until after the spots show up, but they go away within a couple of hours of taking the antronex.

I would also like to recommend water with lemon. It helps keep your liver clean so you can process things better, helping you a stay on top of your allergies. Drink lots of it the water and the lemons are good for so much.

Action Steps

1. Find a Chiropractor in your area who will let you buy Allerplex and Antronex. Go to Standardprocess.com for more information.

2. Drink lemon water every day. Add it to your water right away in the morning. You want to drink at least one ounce of water for every 2 pounds of body weight, or ½ your body weight in ounces. If you weigh 100 pounds that is 50 ounces of water, work up to your recommended amount by drinking a little more every day.

Summer Foods

Summer is a great time to detox. You don't even have to do anything weird. Go to your local farmers market and stock up on whatever is fresh. Avoid processed foods and sit outside in the fresh air whenever you can. Your lungs are one of your body's primary filters so breathe deeply, there you go you are detoxing.

I like to throw together huge salads fresh greens, tomatoes, cucumbers, and whatever else is available. Throw in some herbs, olive oil, salt and pepper and you are all set to go. Add some chicken from the grill and you have a complete meal.

Another thing to keep in mind at the farmers market is honey. Fresh local grown honey tastes wonderful, and it's better for you than store bought. There is research showing that local honey will help prevent allergies, because it is made with the pollen your body is fighting.

Now I put this under summer foods because I live in Michigan, and we only get fresh stuff in the summer and fall. If you are lucky enough to live somewhere that has good weather. Go all the time.

Action Steps

1. Find your local farmers market, and check it out.

 2. If you are concerned about allergies get some local honey.

To much Sun

I can't tell you how important drinking enough water is. When our son was little he went over to a friend's house. The mom decided to take them all to the lake for the day.

She packed sandwiches and a juice box a piece. It was a really hot day, and they were in the sun from 11am to 5pm with no water. Cody was sick for days after we got him home.

Now he has to be careful all the time, if he is too hot he gets sick. The heat stroke affects every part of his life he can't exercise like he wants or work outside which he loves unless he pays constant attention. It is so much better to take care of yourself, before you end up with heat stroke, because once you've had it you have to be on guard for it for life.

Sunburns are another issue you have to watch for in the summer. We are told to always put sun screen on our outside, but what could you do inside. We have found consistently that when we are eating, drinking, and supplementing right we don't get burned.

The most important vitamin we take when we are going to be outside is something called Cataplex F. You can get Cataplex F from a

Chiropractor who carries the Standard Process brand vitamins.

We discovered the Cataplex F after a seminar. In an offhand comment the Doctor giving the seminar mentioned that he used Cataplex F to help prevent sunburn. So we decided to do some experimenting and try it the next time we were out.

We were invited to go spend the day jet skiing with some friends, so we each took some before we went and a couple more a few hours into the day. We didn't use any sun screen or anything else.

After being in the sun for almost 8 hours none of us had any burns at all, not only that, but Cody was doing really well no signs of problems at all.

My husband of course is never satisfied that something worked so he went out the next day without taking it. His thought was that he had already been in the sun and he didn't burn so he must be used to it, he was also testing the vitamin to see if it had really worked. He came home with the worst water blistered burn he'd ever had in his life.

Cody had been out with him, but he'd been taking the vitamins all day, mostly because I'd threatened him, but he does have a little more common sense than his daddy.

We never go out without the Cataplex F anymore and we haven't had a sun burn since.

We use either sesame seed oil or coconut oil on our skin in the summer, not chemical sunscreens. It also helps to take it internally cook with it. There is a lot of research out there saying the chemical sunscreens are bad for you, so we choose to avoid them.

You can get natural sunscreens online. We like Vitacost.com it's a great place to pick up vitamins, and other natural things for way less than you would pay at a health store. I've also found some nice recipes online that I use for my family in the summer.

Now you will find some disagreement online about making your own sunscreens, so you really need to do your research and figure out what is best for your family.

A good rule of thumb when doing any research is to follow the money. If the people knocking the home made sunscreen are sunscreen manufacturers of course they don't want you to make it yourself. Take a little personal responsibility here and make an informed decision for your family.

Remember your skin is your largest organ. Yes your skin is an organ. I didn't know that either. If you wouldn't eat something why would you put it in your body through your skin? Your skin absorbs everything. Our rule of thumb is if you wouldn't eat it don't put it on your skin.

Action Steps

1. Always make sure you have enough water in the summer. We like to add extra mineral drops to ours to help as well. Tired of drinking plain water don't forget you can add lemon, or I like to cut up fresh fruit and let it soak in the water over night that way in the morning we have slightly flavored water, strawberries and oranges are our favorites.

2. It's summer eat lots of stuff that's good for you proper nutrition will help protect your skin. Lots of fresh fruits and vegetables, eat them raw when you can to get even more of the vitamin protection.

3. Try some natural oils for sun protection if that suits your family. We like sesame and coconut oils. Remember if you wouldn't eat it, don't put it on your skin.

4. Get some Cataplex F from Standard Process. Remember you have to get it through a Chiropractor.

The Pietri Dish

Well it's time to go back to school, nothing like sending your kids right into a petri dish. For those of you that don't remember science class the petri dish is what they use for growing bacteria.

Dirty handles, runny noses, holding hands in line are all things that add up to sick kids pretty quickly. You know you have about a month before all the things they are exposed to start showing up, and they come home sick. What if you could do something to help improve their immunity before they got sick?

In case you've missed it. The over use of anti-bacterial cleaners has resulted in some super flesh eating bacteria's that we just can't fight. Like Methicillin-resistant Staphylococcus aureus, or MRSA for short, and let's not forget about the new super villain Carbapenem-Resistant Enterobacteriaceae or CRE. So we recommend something that has been used for hundreds of years. That as far as we know doesn't cause these mutations.

We recommend "Thieves Oil" to our patients and use it ourselves. The use of thieves' oil is based on the story of a group of French thieves during the "Black Plague".

The story is told about a band of thieves that were robbing, the dead during the plague. They mostly chose to rob the homes of the wealthy. After all why would you rob poor people? When they were captured the judge offered them a smaller punishment if they would tell how they avoided getting sick. They told the judge about an, oil that they had created a blend of healing oils that they would pour onto the masks they wore over their faces as well as into their skin.

   Now I would recommend you spend a little time online reading about thieves' oil. Just remember that some of the oils in the recipe have been scientifically proven to kill bacterium and viruses.

Here is the recipe I use for my family.

   40 drops organic Clove Bud essential oil
   35 drops organic Lemon essential oil
   20 drops organic Cinnamon Bark essential oil
   15 drops organic Eucalyptus essential oil
   10 drops organic Rosemary essential oil

You mix them all together in a dark bottle. If you don't use a dark bottle the essential oils will react with light and go bad faster. I add a carrier oil to mine. I prefer Sesame oil, but olive oil will work in a pinch. On a personal note my kids find this a little bit too lemony. You can play with the recipe a bit until you get what you like. There are different recipes online, but they all are basically the same core oils. If you aren't into making it yourself, you can buy some premade online, just keep in mind that the premade kinds can get a bit pricey. It is actually cheaper in most cases to buy all the separate oils yourself and make it.   We go through a lot of the oil and at $40 to $120 a 2 ounce bottle, if you buy it premade it adds up really fast.

   I rub a little into my kid's chests before they leave home. You can even send some to school with them in a little bottle, just like any other hand sanitizer; it definitely smells better than the chemical ones.

Action Steps

1. Make or buy some "Thieves Oil" and apply it to your family.

Thieves' oil also smells really good in a diffuser. It's a safe non-chemical way to make your house smell nice.

I also like to spray it on the dog bedding so their area doesn't get smelly.

Colds and Flus

Well you've made it through September and now all the bugs are starting to show up, time to improve your immune system to help keep you healthy. Now I'm not going to say we never get sick, but last year when all the people around us were on their second month of the flu or cold whatever they decided it was. We had only been sick for a couple of days, and not even that sick.

I often forget to get out the Echinacea before we get sick, oops, no one is perfect. You need to start getting that into your family any way you can, nothing I've ever heard of has been proven to strengthen your immune system better.

Echinacea builds up in your system as you take it. The longer you take it the stronger your immune system gets.

My family likes a cold and flu tea from Yogi Teas it has a lot of the things you need in it, add some honey and you are doing great. Honey has been proven to fight bacteria and it's a nice natural sweetener. We always recommend that you drink lots of hot stuff this time of year. The viruses and bacteria like your body to be a certain temperature when they are attacking you, so we try to scald the little beasties to death.

Fenugreek is one of my absolute favorites for fighting the goop that gets in your chest when you have a cold, or anything else. I came across this study when I was researching fenugreek for my family.

"During a three-month winter period, 20 volunteers, 10 with colds and flu symptoms and 10 without, consumed half a teaspoon of fenugreek seeds twice a week in a curry. The cold-afflicted volunteers reported immediate and sustained relief from symptoms of running nose, cough, sneezing, sore throat and fatigue. Volunteers who were fit and healthy at the outset remained that way for the duration of the trial, despite usually coming down with a cold at least once in the same period."

The test was conducted by Anglo-Indian chef Gurpareet Bains, author of Indian Superfood. He plans further clinical trials with the help of an American university.

"We already know that some foods and spices can help alleviate the symptoms of a cold, but the results of these studies show that fenugreek is significantly more beneficial," he said."
This article is from the Times of India website.
Fenugreek has consistently worked well for my family. Fenugreek is also good for insulin control and is recommended for many diabetics. It has a pleasant side effect; it makes you smell like maple syrup.

Another family favorite is licorice root. I take it not only during cold season, but my son and I take it for our asthma. It is an anti-inflammatory, behaves like an expectorant, and helps with dry cough, bronchitis, and asthma.

The root may also help lubricate the irritated and inflamed respiratory tract and sore throat, relax bronchial spasms, and combat viral flu, cold and other respiratory tract infections. You can drink both fenugreek and licorice root as a nice warm tea or you can take them in pill form. The tea form is probably a better choice, once you have a cold, but taking the pill form may help you not get a cold.

Garlic is another family favorite for this time of year. Now I know it's terrible to go around smelling like garlic all the time, but it is so good for your immune system. Garlic is a natural antibiotic, but it is safe and doesn't cause the mutations that the manmade antibiotics cause. If you just add it to your meals it should be enough. That actually brings us to the next step.

My husband and sons favorite choice when they feel a cold or flu coming on is to drink hot sauce right out of the jar. Hot and spicy stuff really does make a difference in fighting off the cold and flu.

Winter is a good time to hit the ethnic isle at the store. Mexican, Italian, Indian foods all have a lot of the spices that will help your body fight viruses and infections during the cold winter months. It's interesting that Ayurvedic medicine believes that when it's cold out you should eat hot and spicy foods and when it's warm out you should eat cooling foods. I think they are right, but no matter how sick I think I'm going to get I can't make myself drink hot sauce out of the bottle.

Another thing we recently discovered was ginger. Ginger breaks up the goop in your throat; it's great for post nasal drip. My husband and I were both going through this symptomology of having goop that we were choking on in the backs of our throats. That was really the only symptom that we were experiencing. It was especially bad at night, keeping me awake. One night when I was sitting there sulking because it was going to be another sleepless night. (I had tried valerian, but it wasn't helping because I was choking not the normal sleepless night.) I pulled out my trusty IPod and began looking for a cure that I had available.

After about a half hour of searching sites for post nasal drip I found one site that mentioned ginger. I got up took two ginger and 15 minutes later I was asleep. I took it for the rest of the week and gave it to my husband it cleared it right up for both of us. It's so nice to have another tool in your cupboard.

Speaking of tools in your cupboard lets talk about one you probably already have. Vicks Vapor Rub is one of my all time favorites. I still get a bit stuffy at bed time even though my allergies are well controlled. So I always reach for the trusty Vicks to help me get to sleep. I was glad when I discovered a new way to use it.

Thanks to all our hard work I do get sick less than I did growing up, but when something comes around I get the sickest. I had a cold, but it was a weird one. I was a bit stuffy and sometimes I felt like my chest was congested but that was all at least during the day.

At night I would cough and cough and nothing I did changed it. We tried a humidifier, sleeping sitting up, all my normal vitamins and teas, I even (gasp) tried cough medicines for the first time in probably 10 years, but nothing would make the coughing stop.

I of course was already layered in Vicks after all it is my favorite, but even that wasn't breaking through the coughing. I was desperate. I had taken to sitting in the bathroom corner so that my coughing wouldn't keep everyone else up. I had my IPod and was surfing the net looking for ways to stop coughing when I stumbled upon a crazy piece of advice.

The web site said to rub Vicks on the soles of your feet and cover with socks to stop night time coughing. I was really tired so it was worth a try. I went back to bed grabbed some socks and covered my feet with Vicks. I added a little to my chest for good measure.

When I laid down the coughing got worse again, but I expected that. After about half an hour it stopped and I fell asleep. I didn't put it on before bed the next two nights to experiment a little, but when I did finally put it on the coughing stopped right away.

My kids seemed to come down with the same virus so we tried the Vicks thing on them immediately. It worked and they did not spend the whole night coughing.

Action Steps

1. Take Echinacea it is one of your best friends when you are fighting the colds and flus. Now most Chiropractors and other health nuts that we know take it year round, I know people that have taken it consistently for 20 or more years and they are never sick.

Now I don't know if it is because I like to give my body a break or if it is because we are cheap, but we do like to take some time off. One thing we recently found out about Echinacea is that when you pour the capsule out on your tongue it should either bubble, burn, or tingle to show it is alive and active.

We like to get our Echinacea from the Standard Process MediHerb line you can get either pill form or liquid and their quality is so good it burns all the way down. We know Standard Process' standards are the absolute highest in the industry in everything they do; I know that if I recommend it, they are not going to let me down.

2. Fenugreek is an Indian spice. You should learn to love Indian food it is very healthy. You will find many of the herbs that I mentioned in almost every dish you get. You can get fenugreek in pill form and it is very easy to take that way. While we always prefer Standard Process for everything we have been pretty happy with the herbs from Nature's Way, while they aren't up to Standard Process standards I would say they come in second and have a nice selection of herbs.

You can also go to an Indian store and get the actual seeds, my husband likes to make tea from them and you can grind the seeds up and add them to your food.

3. Licorice root is another one I get from both Standard Process and Nature's Way. If you can find foods that contain actual licorice eat them. It is hard to find real licorice. Licorice flavoring does not contain actual licorice so that black licorice you were craving probably won't do the trick.

4. Eat foods that are spicy and make you feel warm inside, it's actually very comforting on a cold day. My children have grown up with some very different comfort foods than we did. If you can handle hot sauce drink some at the first sign of a cold, my husband swears it works and so do a lot of his patients. I still can't make myself do it.

5. Try ginger especially if you are dealing with post nasal drip it took care of our problem right away. Ginger is something you can find in both Indian and Asian cuisine.

6. Rub Vicks Vapor Rub on your feet for coughing.

Motion Sickness

Motion sickness is actually something we hear about a lot. It's not a seasonal complaint, but we have been finding a kind of dizziness that seems to go with some of the viruses we have been seeing in the office.

The first thing you need to do with motion sickness is get adjusted. The Chiropractor needs to check your ears and your neck. I have to make a case for Palmer Chiropractic graduates here. They are actually taught the soft tissue adjustment for the ear and I'm telling you right now if that ear isn't right nothing you do is going to fix it. We have seen it too many times in both our family and our patients.

After you have taken care of your neck and ears you need to take ginger root. When my husband was in the military they tried everything they could think of on his motion sickness everything that is but ginger root.

We actually didn't really discover ginger root until after he finished school. The results were amazing for the first time in his life Marty was not only able to ride in the back of the car without getting sick he was able to read and play with the kids. It was amazing. I have to take it too I was always a car sleeper because otherwise I would get sick, I still would rather sleep when traveling, but now when I wake up I feel okay instead of sick.

Action Steps

1. Find a good Chiropractor immediately, emphasis on good. Chiropractic is an art and different doctors have different specialties and strengths. Shop around and don't be afraid to try more than one, you can't trust your health to someone who just doesn't get you.

2. Make sure your Chiropractor can adjust your ears as well as your neck.

3. Stock up on ginger before you travel it's always handy to have. It's also antibiotic, anti-inflammatory, and it's a pain killer. If you can find real ginger snaps or ginger ale with real ginger in it, it will make it a lot easier to get it in your kids.

Reclaim Family Time

When did you become a bad parent if you didn't sign your kids up for every activity that came along? I know people who spend every evening running from activity to activity the only time they spend together is in the car driving to and from events.

They aren't even together then. They have one parent going one way with some kids and the other parent heading a different direction. How can this be considered family time when everyone is stressed out?

The time stealers don't even respect Sundays now. Religious or not we all need some downtime. Our families are lost in a haze of running to and fro.

Think about this. Imagine yourself on your death bed. Are you going to say "Boy I wish I had signed my kids up for more activities" or "I wish we had spent more time being a family" which one?

I actually see all this business as an attack on our families. You have no time at all to install the values you want in your children.

I have helped several of my patients evaluate their busy lives, with great success. The process is simple.

Step 1 Write down all the activities you are involved in, work, school everything it helps to make a list for each person.

Step 2 Write down how many hours a day are spent on work and school for each person. Include travel time.

Step 3 Note how many extra activities is each person in.

Step 4 Look honestly at each activity does it really make the person happy or is it just filler.

Step 5 Show the kids their lists. Ask them to pick the one thing they can't live without, and the one thing they really don't care about.

Step 6 Whittle your way down until your schedule becomes more manageable. Remember this is your family focus on what works for you.

Step 7 schedule down time, if it's not scheduled it will be forgotten. Putting it on the schedule gives it the same level of importance as everything else in your life.

Your family deserves some rest. According to the Centers for Disease Control stress is one of the leading causes of illness. I observed this up close when my husband was in Grad School.

When Marty was at Palmer getting his Doctorate there were days that he was gone from 6am to 1am. The kids would go days without seeing him.

He was working completely on adrenalin. At the end of the trimester he would collapse from the fatigue. Usually it would be a cold that took him out the second he tried to take a breath.

We see this collapse in many of our patients and their families, just when you think you are finally going to have down time some one gets sick.

You have a choice wait until your body schedules your down time. (It will always choose the worst possible time.) Or schedule it yourself, a little time set aside for you and your family every week is a great thing.

Our top 10 herbs

I'm going to give you some basic information on our favorite herbs and why we use them. If you need more information go online and check them out. These are the herbs we reach for constantly, but don't think you have to stop with them.

1. Echinacea contains the Vitamins A, C, and E three of the more important cancer fighting vitamins. While we focus on using it to improve our immune system during cold and flu season it has been linked to helping with some forms of cancer, increasing your white blood cell count, cleansing and strengthening organs like your spleen, pancreas and liver. As I mentioned before you want the Echinacea to tingle and burn a little on your tongue to show that it is active and alive. They have given Echinacea credit for helping with a lot of different things it would be worth your while to look into it.

2. Fenugreek is what we use to help us breath during cold season. Fenugreek seeds are a strong, mucilaginous antiseptic and kill infection of any kind in the lungs. For most of my life every time I got a cold it turned into Bronchitis. In the 10

years I have been taking Fenugreek during cold season none of my colds have turned into anything worse.
I have also heard of Fenugreek being recommended to help mothers with their lactation if they are nursing, as well as people using it to help control their diabetes.

3. Licorice has been a life saver. We recommend it to people with Asthma and Arthritis. Cody uses it for his Asthma like symptoms that he developed from being exposed to mold.

4. Garlic contains Vitamins A, B1, and C, Selenium, Sulphur, Calcium, Manganese, Copper, Iron, Potassium, and Zinc. It dissolves cholesterol, lowers blood pressure, is an antibiotic, kills parasites and has an all-around healing effect on your body. The smell you get from the garlic is mostly the sulphur. Sulphur has a lot of healing qualities, and mosquitos don't seem to like the smell either.

5. Gotu Kola is a supplement we use on days when our brains are feeling tired and behind. Gotu Kola wakes up your brain. Gotu Kola has been shown to help with high blood pressure, cataracts, depression, and mental fatigue.
   I like to drink Gotu Kola tea in the morning there is no caffeine, but it helps you feel awake, and gives you energy.
   I also like to drink it when I'm going to be writing. Some days my brain just doesn't feel up to it, and the Gotu Kola really helps.

6. Valerian relaxes muscle spasms relieving pain. Valerian is what Valium is based on the main difference between the two is if you overdose on Valium you die Valerian should just give you a bad headache.

   Valerian root has been used to treat hives, shingles, some kinds of eye infections, and pain. We like it for nights we can't sleep either from stress or pain. Some reports say you can take it all the time and some reports say you can't I like to err on the side of caution so we don't take it all the time.

7. White Willow is what aspirin is based on. We use it for all the same reasons you would aspirin.

8. Ginger; I told you that we mostly use Ginger to relieve motion sickness and throat congestion, but we also use it for digestion, and weight loss.

   Ginger has warming properties that are nice for someone like me who is always cold. I don't know if it is true, but I like to think it helps with weight loss because of the heat.

9. Cascara Sagrada: (Rhamus Purshiana)
I have heard Cascara Sagrada referred to as "man's best Roto-Rooter". It will normalize severe constipation. While it has a strong laxative effect it's not really a laxative. It stimulates the muscle walls causing contractions and it has amodin in it to keep it in control. We take it when we are starting to feel backed up or I like to take it for a couple of days every other month as kind of a quick detox.

Cascara Sagrada is not considered habit forming and has been shown to normalize your colon over time. It has also been shown to help pass gall stones. As with anything you are going to take talk to your doctor first. I recommend finding a Naturopathic doctor of some kind, Md's know about drugs you want someone who knows about herbs. I don't know how long you can consistently take Cascara Sagrada as with almost all herbs it depends on who you are talking to.

10. Turmeric is a spice found in Indian food and some mustard. Turmeric has been shown to help relieve depression, but it is good for a number of things including weight loss.

One thing I didn't mention was that most of these herbs are anti-inflammatory as well. Meaning taking them helps relieve inflammation in your body, reducing pain. You will find most herbs have some pain relieving qualities.

I have been researching herbs for years and these are the ten my family takes consistently, but there are hundreds I still haven't even heard of you may find a whole different set of herbs helps your family. Your spice rack is a mini medicine cabinet. Adding spices to your food will not only make your food taste better it will improve your health.

Look at your favorite spices and see what they are good for. Look up cinnamon we have quite a few patients who swear it relieved all their pain, and all they did was add it to their toast. Good health does not need to be difficult.

Top 5 Vitamins

Remember not all vitamins are created equal. We always tell our patients to read the labels if you don't know what something is maybe you don't want to put it in your body. Try to find vitamins that are made from natural things like vitamin C from rose hips.

1. B vitamins are our absolute favorite. They help control the crankier members of our family.

You might only show the signs of being low on one, but you should take them all. They are made to work together.

Food is still a great place to get your B vitamins. Standard Process has two great B's that are made to work together. They are Cataplex B and Cataplex G one is your water soluble B vitamins and the other is the oil based B's between the two you have both kinds covered.

2. A Vitamin is important for protecting your body's tissue. It is also good for your eyes and fighting the effects of pollution on your body.

The problem with A is that toxicity is a very real problem. We recommend getting it through your food if at all possible. Good sources include carrots, green leafy vegetables, eggs, and milk. There are other sources, but these are the ones most people have in their home.

3. Vitamin C is a vitamin we should all be familiar with. We know it is good for our immune systems, but did you know it is also good for detoxing your body?

When our son Cody was little he discovered the plastic (Made in China) blinds in his room. We bought them because they said "No Lead". At one of his check ups we discovered that he had lead poisoning.

We went straight from the doctor's office to the store to buy a bottle of chewable, orange flavored vitamin Cs. I spent the whole day giving him "candy" and filtered water.

The next day when we took him in to be retested all the lead was out of his system. We replaced the blinds with good old fashioned shades. No more problems.

Vitamin C is also good for removing excess Vitamin A from your body if you have too much. Make sure you do not buy synthetic Vitamin C always buy vitamins that are made from real foods. Rose Hips are a great source. We actually pick our own if we can get there before the birds.

4. Vitamin E has gotten some bad press in the last few years. The funny thing is when we reviewed the different studies that said it was bad they had all used synthetic vitamins. We absolutely agree synthetic Vitamin E is bad for you.

Vitamin E helps feed the Pituitary Gland, the heart, muscles, skin, and prevents or dissolves blood clots. I use it to help support my heart.

Vitamin E slows down the aging process. It has also been shown to be useful on skin healing scars and in a couple of our patients healing their spider veins. Rubbing E lotions on their legs was the only health change they made.

5. Vitamin D is the vitamin we turn to in the winter. The best place to get it is from the sun. It's free, sugar free, calorie and fat free. You just can't beat the sun as your Vitamin D source.

Good sources any animals that grow in the sun. Vitamin D is higher in summer milk and cheese than winter go figure.

Top Mineral Deficiencies

We forget how important minerals are to our bodies. Minerals are used in almost every reaction in our body. From testing and dealing with our patients these are the minerals we found lacking most often.   I recommend hair testing if you are wondering what you are low on.

1. Chromium is an essential mineral for your body. It helps your body deal with sugars by working with insulin to remove glucose from the blood steam.

2. Zinc is probably more important for men to worry about than women. We have a quick test for zinc deficiency at the office. It's very simple if you are deficient you don't taste anything, and if you aren't the taste is horrible. Of the patients that have taken the test 100% of our male patients have been deficient, and one of our females.
   Zinc feeds most of the tissue in your body, but the big one is the prostate along with spermatozoa. We won't go into the signs of deficiency let's just say men make sure you have your zinc.

3. I recently read a report that said all Americans are low on Magnesium. Magnesium and Calcium go hand and hand. Unfortunately we put Calcium in everything which bonds with and strips your body of magnesium. We recommend that our patients take magnesium lactate not magnesium with calcium. Magnesium is good for your heart and your bodies other muscles.

We have found that our patients who are low on Magnesium have problems sleeping and are prone to Charlie Horses (calf cramps) in the middle of the night.

We have also found them to have a tendency towards constipation. When we recommend Magnesium we have our patients start with 200mgs and work up until they get a loose stool. Once they have reached that we have them return to the level before the loose stool started.

4. Iodine is what they add to salt, in order to stop Goiters. The problem is that the iodine they use isn't really good for people. We choose to use sea salt and get our iodine some place else. The best place to get iodine is seaweed most people use kelp.

Iodine deficiency is easy to test for you simply apply some iodine to your arm and see how long it takes to absorb. If it absorbs really quickly you will want to have a proper test done.

5. Sodium is important. I know we have all been told to watch our salt intake making sodium seem like the bad guy. It's not.

Too little sodium is a danger as well. Sodium works in our blood, without enough your blood will clot, often causing a stroke.

Sodium is responsible for maintaining the proper amount of water in our bodies, keeping us hydrated and letting our bodies do their work. People who seem to sweat excessively for no reason may not have enough sodium in their bodies. This can also be the cause of crying for no reason.

You can actually visually detect low sodium by looking at someone's mouth. If the left corner is lower than the right you are low on sodium. If your right is lower it is potassium.

It is important to remember that potassium and sodium work together.

6. Sulphur is found in every cell in your body, but it is highest in your hair, skin, and nails. That is why some people refer to sulphur as the beauty mineral.

People who are low in sulphur have poor growing nails and hair, along with several skin conditions. Sulphur is needed to work with Collagen keeping your skin youthful and elastic.

Sulphur is what causes the smell when you've eaten eggs, garlic, or onions. It's found in several of those foods that bite back like radishes or horseradish. We like to get our sulphur in eggs because they contain the protein to help it be more effective.

This section was to give you a look at how important minerals are. All minerals work together in a perfect combination.

Think of your body like soup. Who wants soup that's too salty (sodium) or has to much garlic (sulphur)? You want a soup that has all the right ingredients. It's the same for your body your vitamins and minerals are a complex recipe that makes up the soup that is you.

The problem is getting your minerals in a form your body can actually digest. When you can't get your minerals from food we recommend colloidal minerals because they seem to be used in the body best.

Things you should do year round

1. Drink Green Tea. I know I talked about it in the winter blues section, but green tea is good for a lot of other things. Green tea helps support testosterone production so it's good for men. It's been linked to weight loss, mood improvement, anti-cancer, rheumatoid arthritis, lowering high cholesterol levels, helping with cardiovascular disease, and it helps fight infection. It's believed to be important in the long healthy lives in the orient. We love green tea in fact I might need a cup when I get home.

2. Kombucha Tea is a fermented food, kind of like pickles or yogurts. If made wrong it pretty much is vinegar, if made right it tastes like sparkling cider. Kombucha contains the natural probiotics that your body needs to be healthy. It is also very high in B-vitamins. You can read more about Kombucha in my husband book," Tea of Immortality"

3. Chiropractic while this is not a book on Chiropractic, you need to understand that a good

Chiropractor knows about more than just your spine. If you found a Doctor to buy the "Standard Process" vitamins from, he is probably very well versed in nutrition, and may be a good future resource if you have any problems.

4. B-vitamins are important. B-vitamins assist in rebuilding your nervous system and organ repair. Your body burns through B's very quickly. They are depleted even faster when you are under stress so you will want to take them throughout the day. Alcohol depletes B-vitamins and in some cases it can be quite severe.

5. Drink your water! I have a lot of patients who "just can't drink all that water". That is their excuse not to drink any water; they are our sickest and most difficult patients. Dehydration is one of the most pressing problems in this country. This is weird considering Americans have more access to good water than just about any other country. Another excuse is, "It makes me have to pee." Your body will adapt after a while and you will start pushing it out in other places like the lungs, skin and intestines.

   A good test for dehydration is to pinch the top of your hand and see if it pops back to where it is supposed to be or if it just sits there. If it just sits there you are dehydrated.

   Another sign of dehydration is excessive hunger. We have found with many of our overweight patients that when they answer their hunger pains with a glass of water they begin to lose weight. Start drinking your water as soon as you get up eventually you will drink all you need in a day.

Serve water with dinner your kids have been eating who knows what all day and need to do a little interior cleaning as well.

A little plug for water filters here. I'm not going to go into the statistics, let's just say your water isn't as fresh as a mountain stream. Get the best filter you can afford.

You might not get all the chemicals out of your water, but getting some chemicals out is better than none. We like the Zen Water filtration system you can get on Amazon or at their website Zenwateronline.com check both the prices vary.

6. Eat as naturally as you can. The fewer chemicals you find in your food the better. I am not going to say you have to eat all organic, but some organic isn't a bad idea.

Organic food is grown with no chemicals placed directly on them. Our world is very toxic and our bodies just can't keep up, anything you can do to relieve some of the toxic overload has to help. Doing something is better than doing nothing. Every little choice makes a big difference.

Summary

In this book I've shared with you the simple tricks we use to help keep our family healthy. Taking care of your health isn't about uprooting your family and turning your life upside down.

It's a series of small steps a little change here and there can make all the difference. Something as simple as buying organic or unsweetened peanut butter will quickly become a natural part of your life.

The Japanese practice something called Kaizen. Kaizen stands for continuous incremental improvement.

Think about it. If you choose to do just a little better every day, who could you be in a year? What kind of family could you have if every one grew a little, or was just a little bit healthier every day?

Let's take an easy example of a quick change you can make. I told you to buy organic foods. I don't expect you to go out and throw away your food and buy all new. We certainly didn't do that. I looked at what we ate and made a few simple tweaks. I started by replacing our milk and our peanut butter with organic versions.

Each week we'd replace something we ran out of with something better.

It's the same with your time. Reclaim a little bit of time every week, maybe you could spend it sitting down to dinner together. They might fight you on it at first, but your kids will appreciate it.

Taking time to plan ahead is important to surviving anything. Could you take a trip without a plan? No you couldn't. You have to know how much money you can spend, and how long you can afford to be gone. So even if you thought you could just leave and hit the road you would have to plan. Life is no different. We all need a plan.

About the author

Stephanie has been helping her husband Dr. Martin Zahl D.C. run their Chiropractic office since 2003. During the years she has developed an almost obsessive compulsive desire to know how to treat every thing with nutrition.

Starting with her health issues and working their way out Stephanie and Dr. Zahl have been able to help 1000s of patients get better.

Stephanie believes that life is a string of small choices, and each day is a chance to improve.

Hopefully reading this book is a small choice that helps you do better.

Other Books by Zahl Family Publishing

All Books available on Amazon Kindle

Health Books
Dr. Martin P Zahl DC

Tea of Immortality: A Little Secret that has improved health for thousands of years.

Hyper Mind Hyper Body ADHD: My life growing up with ADHD. How I've risen above it, learned some tricks to control it, and embraced what it's meant for me.

Stephanie Zahl

Healthy Living Secrets: 10 Habits for a Healthier Next Year

Children's Books

Stephanie Zahl

Elephant Trunk Tusks Ears Kid's Facts & Picture Book

Do you know Hippos?: Children's Picture book